How to Lose Weight Without Dieting

A Step-by-Step Guide to Getting Slim, Sexy and Healthy Body

Tammy Thomas

Copyright

Terms of Use

Any information provided in this book is through the author's interpretation. The author has done strenuous work to reassure the accuracy of this subject. If you wish you attempt any of the practices provided in this book, you are doing so with your own responsibility. The author will not be held accountable for any misinterpretations or misrepresentations of the information provided here.

All information provided is done so with every effort to represent the subject, but does not guarantee that your life will change. The author shall not be held liable for any direct or indirect damages that result from reading this book.

Contents

Introduction

The world moves at a faster pace than it used to. With technology, things happen instantly and therefore, more things seem to happen all at once.

At work, this or that needs done while somebody else needs our help.

A stay at home parent has to juggle taking children to school, sports, helping with homework and keeping up a house.

By the time things have slowed down, we are exhausted, out of energy and out of time. The day has gone by quickly and tomorrow is almost here.

Many of us want to be healthier but our social life, our home life or our job takes up so much time that we end up eating convenience food or hitting up a drive through.

Although both choices may be convenient, they are far from healthy and it gets frustrating to watch your waistline expand, even if you are not eating that much food.

With busy schedules, we sometimes feel stuck in this cycle and breaking out of it is hard to do. That is where we come in.

By picking up this book, you are ready to end the cycle. You are willing to make changes to your lifestyle that will help you look and feel better, without taking up a lot of extra time or costing a lot of money.

Eating healthy does not mean hours of prep work in the kitchen, nor does it mean following complicated meal plans that require extra shopping and specialty foods.

You can fit healthy and filling meals into your busy day. You can fit exercise into your schedule and we will show you how.

Gone are the days of starvation diets, because we believe that the only way to get healthy is by making changes to your diet and your lifestyle in such a way that your body gets what it needs, from the inside out and thus, the changes will be easier for you to maintain.

No more fad diets, yo-yo diets, or trendy celebrity diets that leave you listless so hungry that you end up binging in the middle of the night.

Our plan consists of easy changes, where you can still indulge in your favorites in moderation, eat tasty and filling foods, and still lose weight!

You will be able to do this without buying an expensive gym membership, or having to devote hours and hours to exercise. We can show you how to add basic fitness moves into your daily routine to help boost your weight loss.

It is possible to lose weight and feel great while doing so. This book is your beginning to a better, healthier lifestyle!

Healthy Bodies Begin With Healthy Minds

Our minds and our bodies are connected so when one is not feeling good, the other one will also not be performing as well as it could be.

Reversely, when one feels good so does the other one. In order to have a healthy body you must also have a healthy mind and a positive mindset.

You have picked up this book because you have a hectic lifestyle and want to lose weight and be healthier but you have not got a lot of time.

When our lives are hectic and frantic, it causes stress.

Stress is a factor in weight gain, which is probably something that you were not aware of.

Weight loss or gain is not always as simple as calorie intake and calorie burning, other things can factor in, such as certain lifestyle habits, genetics and stress.

When we feel stressed, our bodies respond by releasing hormones into our system that prepares us to handle the stressful situation by releasing the same things into our bodies that would be released into our systems if we were in a dangerous situation.

To our bodies, being in danger and stress are the same thing. When in danger, the hormones released are meant to bring about short term changes to our bodies that will help us survive.

The changes are not meant to be there for any longer than necessary, but when we are stressed but the changes are not short term, they stay with us. This is why chronic stress is so dangerous to our health in many ways, one of which is weight gain.

Stress causes our bodies to release cortisol, a hormone, which can slow down your metabolism in large amounts.

With prolonged stress, your body will continue to produce this hormone, which makes losing weight even more of a challenge.

This is a hormone, which is meant to be released short-term but stress causes the continual production of cortisol.

Stress will also have adverse effects on your blood sugar levels and contributes to the storage of abdominal fat, which is the fat that has the highest risk fat.

Stress will cause high blood pressure, which can lead to heart problems that can lead to strokes, heart attacks, or even death.

In order to be healthy, you will first have to manage your stress.

As you can see, stress puts a tremendous toll on the body because our body's reaction to stress is only designed for short-term and the effect that it has over a long-term period is far from healthy.

In addition to the above, stress can also trigger bouts of emotional eating and/or cravings.

The hormones released into our bodies while we are stressed trigger cravings for foods that are sugary, salty, and fatty.

When under stress, we crave those things and so we are more apt to hit up a drive through, grab a few donuts or some pre-packed snacks, all of which are full of processed foods, artificial ingredients, calories, and full of fat.

Emotional eating is often an outlet of stress simply because we are not sure what to do, and we translate that stressed feeling into hunger, even though we usually are not.

We eat to burn off the excess energy that stress causes our bodies to build up.

Getting a handle on your stress will not only make you feel better, but it will help your day go by smoother.

When you can handle stress in a healthy way, you are better equipped to deal with life, either at home or at work.

Things are not as hectic and you do not feel as rushed or as anxious. You will even find that you have time for yourself.

Not only will your days be easier, but also you will boost your weight gain factor by learning to manage your stress as well as reducing your risk for stress related diseases.

Stress is not something that can be avoided, there are deadlines to meet, your child might have gotten hurt, or a car accident could have happened, these are things that you cannot control but you can learn to control your reaction to them.

Simple breathing exercises are the best way to give yourself a break from stress.

If you feel your emotions going high, feel flustered, anxious, or overwhelmed you can take a few minutes to just do some basic deep breathing exercises, which will help boost your oxygen intake, and will help you feel not only refreshed and rejuvenated, but more relaxed as well.

These are a great way to boost your energy if you feel like you are starting to lose your energy during the day, instead of reaching for a candy bar, have some fruit and do about five minutes of deep breathing to make you feel more awake and energized.

Either standing straight up, or sitting up straight in a chair, take a slow, deep breath, filling up with air from your lower belly first so that your chest expands last.

Hold this for a few heartbeats and then very slowly exhale until you have slowly let go of all of the air and as you exhale let all of your muscles relax and go loose.

Imagine as you inhale that you are sucking air in through a straw, so that you are filling with air from the bottom first, then your chest and then very slowly exhale, feeling your chest empty first, then the rest of you.

With each exhale, feel yourself go more and more relaxed. Continue doing this until you feel relaxed and calmer.

Exercise can help you burn off that energy that you store when feeling stressed. So take a walk or take a class in Yoga, Pilates or Tai chi, these are low impact classes that not only help you tone muscles but they help manage stress by incorporating breathing exercises at the same time.

Meditation is a great way to help calm your mind and find your center so that you can go about your day without feeling like stress is weighing on you like a ton of bricks.

Meditation can be traditional, you sitting a room and doing some basic breathing and mind calming techniques or it can be in a more familiar way.

You have probably gone into a meditative state before without realizing it, anytime you find yourself doing something and then realizing that you had tuned out or gone to autopilot, which is a type of meditation.

When you are fully engaged in a hobby and your find yourself so focused on what you are doing that you find that your worries and anxieties have just slipped away, that is meditation.

Pick up the daily crossword, jog, garden, or spend some time daily working on a hobby that you enjoy.

Trust us, the time will be well spent so find time for yourself and for what you enjoy.

You can try meditation with visualization as well. This is when you are meditating and you visualize yourself being someplace peaceful and serene.

The goal is to make the visualization so real, that you respond as if you were, letting the stress melt away.

You are forcing your mind to stop focusing on the things that are causing you stress at the moment and to focus on something pleasant instead.

Several guided visualizations also include PMR or progressive muscle relaxation, which is a guided visualization to relax.

Stress makes us tense up our muscles involuntarily so by using a progressive muscle relaxation guided meditation, you will be walked through guided imagery to relax each and every part of your body.

You can buy CD's to listen to or you can find clips online, youtube.com has a variety of guided meditations with or without PMR to help you.

Try pampering yourself occasionally. Anybody who has ever had a massage can tell you that they feel wonderful afterwards so get a 15-minute massage on your lunch break every now and then to help un-knot up tensed muscles and to help promote a feeling of wellbeing.

When things get stressed and situations often escalate quickly and you have no choice but to deal with it, do not panic.

You will never solve a problem by worrying yourself to the point of nearly having an anxiety attack.

Before you lose your cool, take a five-minute time out. If you find yourself in a situation where you are not making progress and it frustrates you, this could be a project that you are momentarily stuck on or even an argument with a co-worker, walk away for five minutes.

Walk around the building, sit outside for a moment and do your breathing exercises, or go grab cold water.

The point is to take a break so that you can re-focus your mind onto something positive. Take a look at the flowers outside; find a butterfly to watch, just get away from the stressful situation, and find something that makes you smile.

Pull out a picture of your spouse, your kids, or even your pets. Close your eyes, pull up a happy memory, and just re-live that memory for a few minutes until you are feeling calmer.

Think of stress like a pressure cooker, the longer it stays closed, the more pressure it puts on you but if you find ways to release the steam inside – the stress – then the pressure never gets to the point of putting you in danger.

You will still have some stress, we all do, but it will not be to the point of being unmanageable if you learn to keep it tolerable.

You have heard of the phrase "letting off steam," consider it as a great analogy to lowering your stress, you are letting off steam to avoid a buildup off stress.

If you know that you are a stress eater and tend to snack when the stress levels rise, the best way to handle this is by already having snacks on hand, healthy snacks that is.

Avoid hitting up the office vending machines or dipping into the kid's snacks if you are at home.

You can find a variety of easy to carry foods to keep on hand. Sunflower seeds are a great solution, as long as they are in the shell.

Eat them one at a time and you will end up feeling as if you are eating a lot when you are in fact, not.

Do not get the flavored kind, those are high in sodium and you do not need that nor do you need the extra calories. Bring raw veggies and either keep them in a cooler or store in the office fridge.

Reach for some carrots sticks and ranch instead of that candy bar. Gum is a handy solution for some, as long as you do not pop it or blow bubbles, this is especially not acceptable when you are at work!

Sugar free gum will give you a way to chew off that nervous energy without adding calories to your day.

At the end of the day, it is tempting to change into sweats and flop in front of the TV for hours, but that is not really giving you time for you.

Try recording your favorite shows and watch them later, with no commercials or you can watch something with your spouse or even your kids.

Call and catch up with family and friends instead of just sitting in front of the TV. Grab your favorite beverage and a good book and head to the porch or patio, or even just to your favorite chair and get lost in the story.

If you have a dog, take your dog to the park or have a play session in the yard, if you have a cat, spend some time petting the cat, grooming the cat or playing with the cat.

The idea is to do something that is meaningful and fun for you instead of just tuning out and watching a TV show simply because it was on and you were tired and bored.

Starting With the Basics

Diets are not easy. Exercise regimens are not easy. It is easy to begin one and then to just stop or taper off.

It is hard to maintain your motivation and your willpower, especially if you make many drastic changes that you must keep up all at once.

By keeping the basics in mind and slowly making changes, we are helping you build up a healthy lifestyle that will be easy for you to maintain.

First of all, you have to want to change. If you are making changes to appease a spouse, then you will not succeed.

This is your life and your health; you are doing this for you and not for somebody else. They could be a factor as to why you are making the changes, but the bottom line about why you are making the changes should be because you want to.

Change must begin with you and only you can maintain the drive to keep up. Unless you are looking forward to making these changes and have a positive attitude about them, you will not succeed.

Consider how good you will feel when you reach your goal every time you feel temptation whispering in your shoulder to help curb your cravings.

Everything that you do will be a choice, but you need to make the choices for the right reasons in order for your goal to be met.

Learn to commit and stick to it. You know you need to lose weight, or else you would not have bought this book.

No more waffling around, this is your chance to change yourself for the better, to be healthy and be fit; this is your goal so stop putting it off.

Procrastination does you no good so avoid it, make today the day that you commit to your new lifestyle and do not go back to your old ways. When you make a commitment and do not stick with it, it causes guilt and that will cause stress. Avoid that cycle and stay committed.

Throw away your notion that you must starve yourself to lose weight; yes, that will work but it is not healthy.

Our book is going to help you lose weight while boosting your health at the same time. When you starve yourself, you lose nutrients that your body needs.

There is no point in losing weight if you are only going to do it in such a way that you end up less healthy afterwards as you did before.

Our plan will allow you to eat, no starving and you will not end up missing essential nutrients, in fact, we will be showing you just what to eat more of, to ensure that you are getting the best possible health benefit from your food.

To lose weight, you should be eating roughly between 1500-1700 calories daily.

You can track your calories yourself, or you can use any number of websites or smart phone apps to help track them for you.

Throw away the notion that if you skip a meal, you are helping yourself lose weight because that is one less meal that you are eating and therefore, fewer calories that you consume.

This is false because you usually end up eating more calories at lunchtime to make up for the missing meal or you will end up snacking more. Do not skip meals.

Do not set unrealistic goals. Instead of having one goal of losing fifty pounds, have losing fifty pounds be your target goal, but break that down further into goals of five-ten pounds each.

By having smaller, more realistic goals you are less apt to give up and more apt to stay motivated and on track.

In addition, when you reach each goal, it just makes you feel good and that in itself will help motivate you.

You want to lose weight, cut down on your sugar intake. We realize that cutting all sugar out will be next to impossible and we do not expect you to.

When you cut out everything that you like totally it will only make you more likely to end up binging on that thing later on, out of frustration for having had to have cut it from your diet.

However, sugar has little value nutritionally and contributes to your likelihood of developing diabetes.

Limit your intake of sugar to only occasionally, save your sugary snacks for a special treat, and to be eaten in moderation only.

If you are feeling your energy wan and want a pick me up, pass up the candy and opt for some fruit, the fructose sugar in fruit is a slow releasing carbohydrate and is a much better and healthier option.

Make sure that you are getting enough protein in your diet. Protein will make you feel fuller and helps boost your metabolism to burn more fat.

Make sure that you are eating a lean protein; skip the greasy and deep-fried foods or fatty cuts of meat.

Watch your fat intake also; about 25% of your daily calories should come from fat, no more than that.

Fast food is usually laden with grease and fat; pass it up for healthier choices. Switch out the cheese you usually eat for low-fat cheese, switch to low-fat or non-fat milk, and look for low-fat salad dressings for a start.

You would be amazed at how much fat you can cut from your diet just by changing out a few foods for non-fat or low-fat options.

Any time that you are moving, you are helping burn calories. Sitting on the couch does not burn any, but even a few trips around the house will burn calories.

You want to lose weight then you need to get moving, simple as that. Even with a busy lifestyle, adding some exercise in is easier than you might think, it does not have to be a long session, but throughout the day, there are ways to sneak in some activity to boost that weight loss factor.

Do not obsess over your scales. Weight yourself at the beginning of each week; do not weigh yourself daily, which will only make you feel as if you are not getting anywhere.

Avoid that frustration and just weight yourself once a week. When you start to lose weight and tone up, it will show because your mirror will reflect it and your clothes will be looser.

No diet plan that has you shedding more than two pounds a week is healthy. The maximum that anybody should ever be losing in a week is two pounds and one pound is the recommended target for healthy weight loss.

This is a slow process but it will help ensure that the weight that you lose will stay off instead of creeping back on.

That is one of the main problems with fad diets, you may shed the pounds fast, but they come back just as quickly.

Workouts That Fit in a Busy Schedule

Dieting helps you lose weight, eat less calories than you burn is the simplest way to explain how dieting works.

If you want to boost your weight loss, you not only eat fewer calories but you should burn more calories as well.

Not only will exercise help you lose weight, but also it helps you tone, strengthen, and get in shape so it has tremendous health benefits.

Dieting works, but dieting and exercise works even better which is why we recommend that you do both, and really, our diet plan is not a diet, because you will not be depriving yourself, you will just be making better choices about what to eat.

Many people feel that in order to have exercise be effective that they must spend an hour a day at a gym, using home gym equipment, or jogging/running and face it, in today's fast-paced life; it is hard to find that sort of time.

This book was designed for you, somebody with a busy schedule but somebody who still wants to get healthy, fit and lose weight but without sacrificing a lot of time.

You do not have to make a daily commitment to a gym. Forget about filling your spare room or garage with home gym equipment, you can find time to lose weight and get healthy.

If you can afford a gym membership, or some home equipment, even just a treadmill, it will be helpful, but not everybody can afford that, so our book is focused on getting fit, without major equipment.

No matter if you have home equipment, belong to a gym or are just wanting to get fit, you will need to find some time to dedicate to working out.

The good news is that it is probably less time than you are anticipating. Like we stated above, you do not have to dedicate hours daily to your workouts.

When combined with sensible eating, working out for around thirty to forty-five minutes three times a week is all that you need to help your body shed pounds quicker than dieting alone.

This will help you lose fat, burn calories, build muscle, and tone your body. Either dieting or exercise alone will help, but in order to get healthy and fit while not having to stress about finding time to do both, by mixing our diet tips along with your easy to do and easy to find time for workouts, you will be getting double the benefits.

Working out three times a week for thirty to forty-five minutes, which is a reasonable amount of time and something that even the busiest of people can fit into their schedule.

You can even break up that into smaller chunks of time, into a workout of ten to fifteen minutes five to six days a week.

Now, there really is no reason why you cannot find at least ten minutes to get your heart rate up and your body in motion for that length of time.

Stop using time as an excuse to delay getting healthy. As long as you get your heart rate up to your target heart rate, then that activity is beneficial to your body and your health.

Everybody can find ten minutes a day, especially if you are motivated to begin losing weight and since you have picked up this book, you are most likely serious.

When are you doing shorter workouts, you need to make sure that they are medium to high impact workouts, if you can combine strength/resistance and cardio, that is even better, exercises like rowing or swimming for example. Even raking leaves is a workout, as long as you pick up the pace.

Exercising consists of two main types:

Strength/Resistance and Aerobic/Cardio. Aerobic exercise-cardio-helps you burn fat, burn calories, build stamina, build endurance, and improves your health, especially your heart.

Cardio is the most efficient way to burn fat and calories. Strength/Resistant training is for toning and building muscle.

The effectiveness of exercise can be measured by your target heart rate, which is the heart rate that you want to achieve to help meet your fitness goals.

Too low means you are not working hard enough and the workout will result in slower weight loss and too high could mean you are putting your heart at risk.

To find your target heart rate, you must first know what you maximum heart rate is; to do that you subtract your age from 220 if you are a male and subtract your age from 226 if you are a female and that is your maximum heart rate.

If you are doing a low-medium impact workout then your target heart rate is going to be between 50-60% of your maximum heart rate.

To boost your weight loss you can use a target heart rate of 60-70%. If you are out of shape and have not exercised in a long time, start at 50% and slowly work yourself up as your endurance builds up. Do not overdo it. Do not push it.

A good piece of equipment to get would be a stability ball or resistance bands. Both come with simple workouts and you will be able to combine your cardio and your resistance workout in one.

You can buy hand weights or you can even use half gallon or gallon milk containers filled with water or sand as home weights.

You might be surprised at what you can do in ten minutes to get your heart rate up to your target heart rate.

Working outside is a great way to burn calories, mowing the lawn, raking leaves, etc. all can bring your heart rate up to your target heart rate.

Cleaning the house, washing your car, and re-arranging furniture in the house can also burn calories and raise your heart rate to that target rate.

Instead of doing your chores at a casual pace, pick up the speed a little. Do you own a dog? Instead of a slow stroll through the neighborhood, take a fast walk and do double the distance, your dog will enjoy the exercise as well.

If you have kids, engage them in a game of tag or take them for a ride. A game of Frisbee or any of your favorite games that you can play, such as basketball, tennis, football or soccer will also make a great workout.

Ten minutes of short play, with or without your friends or family playing will be great way to have a short cardio workout.

You can kick a soccer ball into the net, practice your footwork, same with basketball and tennis, you can always bounce the balls against a wall or your garage door.

No matter if you are starting with a longer exercise period, or a shorter one, you should always have a warm up period first and a cool down period after.

The warm up is to get your heart rate up slowly, and not all at once, towards your target heart rate, to warm up and stretch your muscles and to prepare your body for the upcoming workout.

The cool down helps you ease out of the workout, slowly bringing you target heart rate back down and keeps your muscles from cramping up suddenly like they would if you were to suddenly stop while at your target heart rate.

If you are doing a thirty-minute workout then your warm up and cool down should be about ten minutes long each.

For the ten minute workout your warm up and cool down should be about one minute long each. You can do stretches, slow walking, etc. anything that gets your blood moving about, your heart rate up and

Some basic exercises that can be done at home without equipment are:

Jogging in place

Walking – you should be walking fast enough to get to your target heart rate

Pushups

Sit ups and crunches

Lunges

Squats

Jumping jacks

Shadow boxing

Leg lifts

Walk up and down the stairs

You can use homemade weights or small dumbbells to do curls, to hold while doing squats and lunges to help boost that fat burning power.

Workouts That Can Be Done While at Work

Most of us have to work in order to get by. No job means no bills get paid and so work becomes a driving force in our lives, a very necessary one, and one that occupies most of our day.

Our jobs not only provide us with money, but with stress as well.

Exercise has many benefits, one is to get us fit and healthy and the other one, and it will help relief stress.

That is right, you might have been avoiding exercise because you think that trying to find time to get some workout time into your already busy schedule might cause you stress, but the opposite is true.

By finding time to exercise, your stress level will actually drop. Not a bad extra on top of helping you lose weight and improve your health.

When you have a demanding job, finding time or the energy to get in even a ten-minute workout can be a challenge, let alone thirty minutes.

However, there are all sorts of ways that you can sneak in some fitness at work, helping you release some of your stress and perhaps even leave some free time for when you get home for you to do something fun or have some time with the family.

Few employers will allow you to lug an exercise bike or other gym equipment, but there is one piece of fitness equipment that they probably will allow an exercise or stability ball.

Stability balls might be the better choice for an office because they are filled with sand to prevent them from rolling, exercise balls have no sand and require extra balancing.

By replacing your office chair with one of these, not only will you have to sit up straight, so it helps your posture, but also you will be working and toning your core muscles the entire time you are sitting on it because you will be working to balance yourself.

You can also use the ball to get in some crunches on your lunch break or some other basic exercises but just by using the ball in lieu of a chair, you will reap the benefits of it.

If you live within a few minutes of your workplace, help yourself and the environment at the same time and consider walking or riding a bicycle to work on the days where the weather is good.

If you take the subway, get off one stop before or one stop after your normal stop and walk the difference.

If you are not a morning person, and face it, not many of us are, you can do this at the end of the day only, a walk will often help clear your head of all of the stress and worry from that day and make it easier for you to switch gears when you get home for being able to enjoy your time off.

If you drive to work, stop driving around the parking lot looking for the closest spot, park in the furthers corner of the lot and walk. If you park in the parking garage, park towards the top and take the stairs instead of the elevator.

Unless you work in a high-rise building, consider always taking the stairs instead of the elevator if you are only going up a few flights of stairs.

Instead of emailing that co-worker or using the intercom, get up, walk over, and have the conversation with them at their cubicle or desk. Stop using technology as a crutch to stay in your desk.

Every hour take a small break, not only will this help your eyes from getting computer strain, but it will help your stress and if you use the break to walk around the office, or around the building once or twice, it will help your fitness as well.

You can download free programs from online that will remind you every hour or every two hours to take a small break. Take the long way to the bathroom, or even go down the stairs or up a flight to use a bathroom on a different floor.

Split your lunchtime into halves – take the first half to walk around the area where your office is. Get your co-workers involved, chances are that some of them will be willing to be lunchtime walking buddies with you; leave a pair of sneakers in the office so you are not walking in your office shoes.

Walking is an excellent exercise and will be low impact enough that when you return to the office that you are not a sweaty mess.

Use the last half of your lunchtime to actually eat lunch. If you tend to work through lunch, hunched over your desk, trying to eat and focus at the same time, stop.

There will always be times when you will need to give up your lunch in order to get something important done but do not let it become a habit.

Taking a walk at lunch will allow your mind to clear and getting out of the office and getting your blood flowing can help you think of solutions that you may not have thought of before.

When you are exercising, your heart rate increases, you breathe faster and your blood oxygen levels increase, this will not only give you a mini energy boost, but will give you clarity as well.

A list of simple exercises that you can do in your office:

Sitting straight up in your chair with your feet on the ground, lift your toes, keeping your heels on the ground. You can also do this exercise while standing.

Stand in front of your desk, a chair that does not roll or any piece of stationary furniture, using the furniture to balance, rise up on your tiptoes, lifting your heels off of the floor and then slowly lowing them back down.

Sit in your chair with your back straight and your chin up and raise your left leg up so that it is level with your hip, hold this for as long as you can and slowly lower your leg; repeat with the other leg.

Here is a good one for helping ease some tension if it has built up in your neck and shoulders. Sit up in your chair, or stand up straight and without moving your head, raise your shoulder up to your ear and hold it for several seconds and then do the same with the other shoulder, repeat this about five-ten times per shoulder.

Another good one to relief the muscles from sitting, sit straight in your chair and put your right hand on the backside of your right hip and then slowly twist to the right and hold for a few seconds. Repeat this, going to the left.

This one is great for when you feel the strain of staring at a computer monitor all day, sitting up straight in your chair you will drop your chin to your chest and roll your head to the right, then back to center and then to the left.

Healthy Eating While at Work

When you work long hours and deadlines are looming and there just does not seem like there is enough hours in the day you are looking for food choices that are fast, easy to eat and require minimum preparation.

You want food that is convenient and that will not take up much of your busy day either to obtain or to eat.

However, all of those convenient fast food restaurants, those pre-packaged meals from the local convenience store and the endless choices of frozen foods, ready to zap in the microwave are, with rare exception, far from being healthy.

This is our guide to help you learn how to make healthier choices when at work; remember, we are teaching you to eat smarter, not just eat less and that is why our plan will work.

Any good diet plan will tell you that you must drink water, at least six to eight glasses a day. As a matter of fact, you should drink that much water daily regardless if you are on a diet or not.

Your body works better when it is hydrated, and when you are in a weight loss mode, you need to keep your body hydrated and working properly.

Long days mean that probably tend to reach for drinks that have caffeine in them, but you need to be replacing the majority of those drinks with water, for a different twist on water, try drinking sparkling water instead.

We mentioned this before, but do not skip breakfast. Skipping breakfast will only increase your chances of snacking, usually on junk food, or overeating at lunchtime so you do not do yourself any favors by skipping breakfast.

Your body needs fuel to work, and if you are a busy person, then you need fuel the most, you are skipping the meal that would actually work better towards keeping you energized and alert.

Breakfast does not have to be complicated, you can keep instant yogurt, oatmeal, cereal, and low-fat milk at the office, all of those are simple things that you can eat at your desk.

Fruit is an important part of the diet, not only is fruit full of nutrition and antioxidants, but it makes for a great healthy snack and the sugars in fruit break down better in your body than sugary junk food, making it a great way to give your body a boost.

When you are starting to feel hungry, grab a piece of fruit for a snack and pass up on the office vending machine.

When you have no choices that are healthy at work to eat, you will end up eating unhealthy food instead.

The solution is to keep a selection of easy to prepare foods for you at the office for your breakfasts, snacks, and lunches. One shopping trip a week to keep your office and your office fridge stocked for you to have healthy eating choices is all that it takes.

That will fit nicely into your busy schedule, no waking up extra early to prepare fancy food that you must then re-heat at work.

Some handy things to add to your grocery list to keep at the office are: high fiber cereal, low fat wheat thins or crackers, whole-wheat pitas, whole wheat bread, peanut butter, granola, microwavable low fat soups, dried fruit, nuts, fruit, low fat mayo, mustard, tuna, pre-cooked chicken breast, low fat cheese, lettuce, yogurt, bagged salad, low fat salad dressing, low fat cottage cheese, hummus, deli lunch meat (non-prepackaged).

You can mix and match the above to makes a variety of great lunches and snacks, if you do not have a refrigerator at work, invest in an insulated lunch bag and just bring what you will eat that day.

You can take about five minutes the night before to bring what you need for that day small plastic containers or Ziploc bags that will keep things fresh in your lunch bag all day.

If you do eat out, eat out sensibly. Avoid things that are fried. Substitute a turkey patty or a garden patty for hamburger, skip the cheese, and use mustard instead of mayo.

Restaurant salads are not usually healthy, so much has been added to them that their calorie count is often as high as, or higher than most of the meals.

You can always eat half and save the other half for tomorrow, or for dinner. There are no rules that say that you must clean your plate.

Avoid foods that are smothered in sauces and opt for a side of fruit instead of a side of fries.

Stay at Home Parents Guide to Weight Loss

People that do not stay at home all day to watch kids often do not understand that a stay at home parent does not have free time on their hands all day.

When awake, kids are on the go, usually leaving a wake of destruction in their path.

We understand that even though you are home all day, your day is packed and you have little time for yourself and little time to focus on trying to lose weight.

As a stay at home parent, your first line of defense against gaining weight is to watch your food intake.

Watch what you eat and make healthier food choices for yourself. When you are at home but your attention is on several different things at once, eating is not really a priority and you tend to grab what food you can, when you can, which will never allow you to lose weight and can even cause you to gain it.

Try to keep your calories between 1500 and 1900 to lose a pound to two pounds a week. You can find online calorie counters, track it yourself, or you can add an app to your cell phone.

By tracking your food and beverage intake, you can see what patterns emerge for where the bulk of your calories are coming from and then you can make the necessary changes.

As a stay at home parent, you might be tempted to eat the same things that you feed your children, but remember, they are children and their metabolisms are faster, they are more active and they will burn off the calories faster than you ever will.

When fixing them a grilled cheese, fix yourself a turkey, tomato, and lettuce sandwich on wheat while their grilled cheese is cooking.

Avoid eating the leftover macaroni and cheese, save that for their lunches tomorrow and have yourself a salad with some pre-cooked chicken breast on top for protein.

Fix only enough breaded chicken nuggets for their lunch, fix yourself a bowl of low-fat soup instead.

Avoid their sugary breakfast cereal and opt for a healthier choice, add some banana or other fruit to the cereal to add some extra flavor and texture.

Skip the peanut and butter and jelly for yourself and have some tuna with low fat mayo on wheat instead or buy some low-fat or wheat tortillas and make yourself a wrap sandwich with deli meat, mustard, lettuce and low fat cheese.

Although you might run yourself ragged around the house trying to keep up with your child, or children, unless you get to that target heart rate, you are burning calories, but not as efficiently as you could be.

Turn exercise into a family affair, both you and the kids will benefit from it. If you have a baby or a toddler, put them in a stroller and go for a fast walk, with them in the stroller you do not have to worry about them trying to keep up.

If you have older kids, they can ride their bikes alongside of you. Active parents will tend to raise active kids, give your kids the room and the time to play outside and not be shut in the house, in front of the television.

Childhood obesity is a very real threat to children that are not active enough, so a daily trip outside will benefit everybody.

If all of your children are old enough to ride bikes, go for a bike ride with them. Do not just sit on the front lawn and watch your kids play, be involved.

Get them interested in sports, take them to the park with a soccer ball, softball equipment, or even just to play a game of tag.

When was the last time you played tag with your kids? You would be surprised how winded you get, it is a workout all in itself.

A lot of stay at home parents with multiple children seem to always be in the car, picking up and dropping off children and the temptation to swing through a drive-thru and grab kid's meals for everybody is tempting.

Save the drive-thru meals for special treats for the kids instead of an everyday thing. You can always keep tuna salad, chicken salad, and deli meats on hand for fast lunches.

Soup and grilled cheese is also a fast and filling meal for kids. You should be giving your kids a well-balanced meal as well, making sure they get enough fruits and vegetables in their diet.

When your kids see you eating healthier, it will make them more apt to do the same thing, if they never see you eat fruit, why should they?

When your kids are napping or off at school and you do have some time to watch television, that is fine, but you can turn television into a great way to sneak in several mini workouts.

Find your show, sit to watch it but every time a commercial comes on, get up, and do something! Your goal is to have a few minutes of moderate activity to get your heart rate up to that target heart rate.

Some ideas are to jog in place, take laps around the dining room table, go up and down the stairs, jumping jacks, sit-ups, push-ups, lunges, squats, or use hand weights.

When the show comes back on, sit back down. Next commercial, get back up and pick something else to do while the commercial is on.

It does not matter what exercise you do, just as long as you are doing something. This will get you a minimum of fifteen minutes of exercise every hour.

House chores will also burn calories, not only do you burn them when running after your kids, but cleaning also burns calories so think of that when you are cleaning and grumping about it, you are doing something that has a double benefit, it will get your house clean and it will help you lose weight.

Instead of sitting in your pajamas or sweats, in the morning put on some yoga pants and a t-shirt, something that you would exercise in to help get you motivated and keep you motivated.

Keep your walking or running shoes by the bed so that they will remind you to do your daily exercises or outside time with the family.

Naptimes are a great chance for you to get in some exercise. You are limited because you cannot go for a walk and leave your kids sleeping.

You should invest in a stability ball, which would come with a workout DVD, or buy or even find online for free workouts for aerobics, yoga or any other at-home work out and use these at home, while the kids are sleeping.

Most routines are about thirty to forty-five minutes long, the perfect amount of time for you to get in your exercise and get a fast shower. You will start to look better and feel better in no time.

Keep some healthy snacks for you to eat during the day. Avoid the chips, cookies and other snacks that you keep on hand for the kids and have fruit or yogurt.

Things to Avoid

This is the section everybody dreads, this is when we tell you what you need to either cut our or limit.

As with anything, if there is something that you crave or love to eat, instead of cutting it out totally just eat it in moderation instead, as a special treat.

Cutting out everything that you love to eat will only cause you to binge on them after so long, so do not deprive yourself, but do limit how much you eat.

Just by cutting down on the foods on this list, you will be cutting back greatly on your fat intake and your calorie intake, which will help you lose weight faster.

The number one thing to avoid is refined sugar. Refined sugar is white sugar, corn syrup, and high fructose corn syrup, which is an ingredient in many beverages, such as fruit juices and colas.

There is no nutritional value to refined sugar and it contributes to your risk of diabetes. When shopping for fat-free foods, check to make sure that corn syrup is not an ingredient, because in some cases, buying the low-fat or regular variety might be the healthier choice, such as with yogurt.

You would be surprised at how many calories, fat and sugars there are in your average serving of condiments.

If you want to lose weight, cut back on your ketchup, mayo, tartar sauces, bbq sauces, sauces in general and most salad dressings.

Mustard has zero calories and is a better choice for sandwiches. Use balsamic vinegar for salad dressings. If you must use condiments, use them sparingly.

You need to cut out fried foods from your diet. Look for foods that have been baked, boiled or sautéed instead of deep-fried.

Pass up the deep fried crispy chicken on your sandwich for a grilled chicken breast instead.

Have the baked fish instead of fish and chips. If you end up at a drive-thru, just get a sandwich, but avoid the fries.

Have roasted or baked chicken instead of fried chicken. Vegetables can be steamed instead of being sautéed with butter for a healthier choice.

You should watch your sodium content so avoid soy sauces, things with MSG or pickled foods. In addition, many frozen meals are very high in sodium, so be cautious when picking these out to eat.

Packed meats are also high in sodium so get meat from the deli counter instead or look for low-sodium packaged meats. Same with soups, look for low sodium.

Switch to whole grain wheat instead of white flour. As tasty as white flour is, it is not healthy so opt for whole-wheat options such as bread, tortillas, pasta, etc.

Nearly all processed snack food that is bread based will contain both refined sugars and white flour so pass up those packaged donuts, pastries, and snack muffins.

Limit your intake of cheese and when you do eat cheese, eat the low-fat variety, especially with cream cheese, butter, and cottage cheese.

You should still eat butter instead of margarine though; just limit how much you use at a time.

Processed meats like hot dogs, sausages, bacon, and jerky are full of nitrates, preservatives and fillers and are just not diet friendly.

Skip these choices and opt for healthier and fresher cuts of meat. There are a variety of tasty all-natural sausages and hot dogs out there that are diet friendly, just keep an eye out and look for products with no preservatives.

Use olive oil or canola oil when cooking instead of hydrogenated or partially hydrogenated oils, or you can even cook with real butter, in moderation.

Skip the after dinner drink, alcohol is laden with calories.

Sugar free foods are marketed as diet friendly but they are actually not healthy so skip the sugar free foods.

Artificial sweeteners used in sugar free foods and diet sodas actually cause you to eat more and they contribute to belly fat gain, which is the worst type of fat because it is the fat type that leads to the most health problems.

Sugar free foods will be full of extra fat to make up for the flavor lost by taking out the sugar so just skip the sugar free foods and skip the diet soda, your body will be much better off.

This is the section where people struggle the most, which is why we said to just eat them in moderation, we understand cutting out sugary snacks is hard.

Cakes, sodas, donuts, cookies, ice cream, bakery goods, and pastries are all in this category. Limit your intake of these to special occasions and do not go overboard.

In the case of ice cream, there are several ice creams out there that are all-natural and naturally contain half the fat of regular ice cream and a half a cup will only have under 200 calories in it.

So keep some ice cream of that kind at home and have a half a cup a night, but make sure it is half a cup a night, that way you are still under your calorie count and you are not depriving yourself of your sweets.

Pass up the sports drinks and opt for water instead. Sports drinks are loaded with sugar and calories because they are meant for the serious athlete to replenish what they have lost.

If you are just doing casual workouts, your sports drink will add as many calories as you just burned off. Drink water to offset the water you have just lost while working out instead.

Fruit juices, you would think that they are healthy, but in reality, most are only partially juice, the rest is corn syrup and artificial flavors.

If you are drinking juice, go for organic and all natural choices, or buy fruit and juice it yourself at home.

When you feel a craving, try to take your mind off of it. Switch gears and maybe go for a short walk to take your mind off of your craving.

Do not just sit so you can think of nothing but the craving. Make yourself busy and your mind will very likely forget about the craving.

Think about how much progress you have made and how happy that has made you, keep up the motivation and tell yourself how great it will be to reach your target goal.

If all else fails, try to satisfy the craving with something else or by having that item in moderation only!

If you are a chocolate lover, keeping a few Hersey's Kisses or mini candy bars around is a great way. You are feeling a chocolate craving that will not go away, have one or two of the small pieces of candy only. Chances are that it will be enough to make the craving go away and you will not have added too many calories.

You can also limit craving by making sure that you never are feeling super hungry. Cravings come on when you are hungry so keep your body satisfied throughout the day and your amount of cravings will lessen.

Have a small snack every couple of hours to keep those cravings at bay so when you do start to feel a craving have a yogurt, some fruit, a sparkling water, granola or some trail mix.

Do not wait until you are already hungry, small, light snacks that are healthy are the way to go to avoid the cravings from rearing their ugly heads. Nuts are a great snack because they have protein, which helps you feel fuller.

Keeping Up Your Motivation

Motivation is hard to keep up, especially if you have done so well and then you hit that plateau where no matter what you do, your weight loss stalls.

That plateau is normal and everybody hits it, just like everybody has days where the diet is harder to maintain than or the motivation to exercise is harder to muster up.

Your desire to want to lose weight is your biggest motivator. That desire has already led you to buy this book; it has already manifested itself into prodding you into action.

You know you want to lose weight and you know the reasons why, every time you feel like you might want to give up, remember those reasons.

Write them down and keep a list if it helps you, but keep those reasons in mind, they prompted you into action once, let them keep doing so.

Break your weight loss goals into smaller goals, such as losing ten pounds, then another, then another until you reach your target weight.

This makes your goals more realistic and easier to achieve. When you achieve each goal, that feeling of satisfaction and progress will help keep you motivated and going.

When you are overweight and you have your weight loss target as losing fifty pounds, that seems like a lot, it can be hard to be motivated when you have only lost five or ten pounds, but if your goal for the next three months was to lose ten pounds and you do so, then you have achieved a goal and onto the next goal!

At each goal that you meet, reward yourself. Treat yourself to a massage, a new book, a new gadget, a game of golf, a haircut, a pedicure or even with a food treat, like your favorite candy or a meal at your favorite restaurant, get something that you have not gotten since you started dieting.

When you reward yourself at the smaller goals, you have something to look forward too and it makes it seem all the more worthwhile to stay motivated.

Be proud at every smart choice. If you choose a healthy option over your favorite non-healthy option than congratulate yourself and make a mental note that you have just done something to be proud of.

Never stop taking your healthy choices for granted, because it is not easy to choose healthy over not healthy.

Take a few seconds to feel proud of yourself at the end of every workout or each healthy choice that you do.

Your body changes themselves will be a great motivation. As your clothes begin to get loser, you will feel better and you will be happy because that is a visible sign that your fitness and diet plan is working.

There is no better feeling than the feeling of satisfaction of putting on clothing and finding that what once was tight is not loose.

Make a spreadsheet of your starting weight and once a week weigh yourself and right down the number.

As you see the numbers start to go down, you will be reminded that you have made these changes for a reason and that they are working, and when you see that they are working then it helps keep you motivated.

Join on on-line support group or even just find other people locally that have the same goal, maybe other co-workers, or other stay at home parents that have the same goals and struggles as you do.

You can help keep each other motivated and celebrate each person's victories together. Everybody can use a little bit of support and encouragement, so make sure that you find people that can help you out with both.

As you lose the weight, make sure that you either get your clothes tailored so they fit, or get new clothes.

By wearing the loose, baggy clothing, you might feel better about losing weight, but when you look in the mirror you will see somebody wearing poorly fitting clothing, and that is not good for your self-esteem.

To avoid that, either donate the clothes that are too big to goodwill or have them tailored so that they fit, when you look good, you feel good.

Do not go around wearing your old fat clothes that no longer fit. Yes, the fact that they no longer fit is great, but you do yourself no favors by wearing them because it does not make you look good.

As you wear clothes that fit, you will not only be aware mentally that you have lost the weight but you will be looking better and better as you keep losing it and wearing clothing that fits your new shape.

You are doing this to look good, so make sure you look good. If it does not fit, donate or have it tailored, do not keep a closet or a box of "fat clothes."

By keeping the clothes that are too big it is like telling yourself that you have a safety net in case you fall of the wagon with your weight loss.

You do not want a safety net because you are not going to fall off the wagon, so do not save your clothes for "just in case." This is a permanent change there is no just in case.

Simple Breakfast Ideas

Eating breakfast provides your body with the energy that it needs to get your day started.

Think about it, you eat dinner and you go to bed, and if you wait until lunch, that is a lot of hours in between, especially if you are a busy person, your body needs something besides just coffee to run on.

Skipping breakfast is a huge mistake to make, especially if you are busy and on the go. Your breakfast choices should include something with protein, which will help fill you up and something that is high fiber, such as whole-grains and fruits.

High fiber foods also help you feel full, so you need to eat less than you would if you were eating something that was not high in fiber.

High fiber foods are a great way to feel full, eat fewer calories, and give your body the energy it needs to start off the day.

Breakfast is important because it gives our metabolism a boost, actually speeding it up slightly after not eating all night so that instead of storing calories as fat, you burn them off faster and more efficiently.

Eating breakfast will prevent you from overeating later on during the day. Breakfast also provides our bodies with much needed nutrients and energy, which we need during our busy days, it increases our attention span, improves our ability to concentrate and can even help with stress, those who have eaten breakfast are usually better equipped to deal with stress as it comes up.

By choosing to eat healthy, you can actually increase your food intake and get much more health benefits than your normal breakfast.

Two multi-grain waffles with some fruit on top and some light syrup along with a cup of low fat yogurt will keep you more energized than a bagel with cream cheese, and it will fill you up more so than a bagel will.

Swap out your white bread for whole grain wheat bread. Use whole grain waffles instead of regular if you buy frozen waffles.

You can find whole-wheat bagels and English muffins as well. Switch out your regular peanut butter for natural peanut butter or better yet, almond butter.

These are just a few ideas, here are some other breakfast ideas that you can mix and match to suit your taste and your needs, and these will make tasty snacks as well.

Use low-fat or non-fat milk instead of whole milk or use soy milk or almond milk instead

Toast some whole wheat bread and spread natural peanut butter or almond butter on top, you can even add sliced bananas and drizzle of honey

Swap out your sugary-sweet cereal for high fiber cereal choices, add in fresh fruit such as strawberries, blueberries or sliced bananas or even dried fruit and sliced almonds

Low fat Greek yogurt mixed with any fruit of your choice

Low fat Greek yogurt mixed with granola and some organic honey

Make your own orange juice or when you buy orange juice at the store, look to make sure that what you are buying is 100% whole orange juice and have a glass with breakfast. Any juice that you buy should be 100% whole fruit, if not, do not buy it.

Try green tea instead of coffee in the mornings, if you need to sweeten the tea, use organic honey. The problem with coffee is that so many do not drink it without adding sugar and creamer, both of which will add extra calories that add up fast. If you drink coffee, try to use as little sugar and cream as you can and limit yourself to a cup a day, if you need more caffeine, drink green tea instead or regular tea.

Scrambled two eggs using just a little bit of butter and serve with whole-wheat toast or a whole wheat English muffin. Eggs are the perfect breakfast food, they are full of protein, and they do not take long to cook. You can scramble them and then use whole-wheat toast or a whole wheat English muffin, along with some Canadian bacon or some turkey bacon and some low fat cheese to make a tasty breakfast sandwich. You can use whole-wheat tortillas to turn some scrambled eggs, low fat cheese, and some salsa into a breakfast burrito.

Make a quick omelet using two eggs and some fresh onion and bell pepper and tomato, or any other topping that you might like along with either whole-wheat toast or a whole wheat English muffin. Fresh spinach and chopped tomatoes makes for a great omelet.

Toasted whole wheat English muffin with some low fat cottage cheese topped with some sliced tomato. You can also top the toasted muffin with low fat cheese and tomato slices and have a hard-boiled egg with it on the side.

Oatmeal, either plain or topped with fruit

Multi-grain or whole wheat frozen waffles

Whole grain bagel topped with some almond butter or natural peanut butter

Fruit makes a great side dish to any breakfast item

Simple Lunch Ideas

Lunch is the meal that helps us get through our day, it should be a balanced meal with protein, and carbohydrates that will help us get through the day.

Eating a balanced lunch will help fill you up and prevent you from tending to snack too much towards the end of the day.

The best way to ensure that you have a healthy lunch is to bring your own. You can make endless sandwich combos with whole grain bread, pita bread, and whole-wheat tortillas to make wraps with.

Your meat that you use should be lean proteins such as sliced egg, tuna, low fat cheese, or lean meat such as grilled turkey or chicken.

You can add any variety of lettuce, spinach, basil, bean sprouts, cucumber, onion, tomato, bell pepper or other vegetable filling to make your sandwich taste better and be more filling.

Opt for mustard instead of mayo or if you must use mayo, just use a little bit and make sure that you are using light mayonnaise not regular. Light ranch or light honey mustard also makes for a great sandwich condiment so just use them sparingly.

When you do eat out for dinner, only eat half of what you order and save the other half for lunch the next day.

That means that a high calorie dinner will make two meals and the calories are far more sensible when spread out between two meals than if you ate the entire meal.

If you eat a balanced breakfast and lunch, then you will not need to eat as much for dinner. Indeed, dinner should be your smallest meal because you are less active after eating dinner than you are after eating breakfast and lunch, so make breakfast and lunch your bigger meals of the day.

You can use your time on the weekend to cook ahead, make a pot of chicken noodles soup to bring for that week or mix up chicken salad sandwiches or tuna ahead of time.

You can cook rice and black beans or other type of beans ahead of time and use as an easy to heat up side dish or combine with some grilled chicken and wrap in a whole-wheat tortilla for a burrito.

Salads are a great lunch for when you are working. You can use a variety of lettuce and salad greens, along with sliced hard-boiled egg, grilled chicken breast, turkey breast, sliced or diced vegetables, and some low fat salad dressing.

Have a fruit or eat it with some pita bread and some hummus on the side.

Low fat and low sodium soups make for a great and easy to carry lunch item. Keep some on hand at the office and enjoy with some cottage cheese or half of a sandwich.

If you are working late and need something more filling with a snack a cup of soup will be a great thing to choose.

You can also find several frozen meals that are geared towards diets, but keep an eye out on the sodium content, as several of them are very high in sodium.

The meals are not usually very large so pair one with some fruit, some yogurt, cottage cheese, or a small salad to make sure that you are full.

Simple Dinner Ideas

Your dinners should be well-balanced, low fat and low calorie but they should also be tasty, flavorful, and filling.

Diets have a bad reputation for being anything but tasty, flavorful, and filling but by just making a few adjustments you can have a balanced dinner that does not skimp on the taste or the flavor.

Your dinners should always include a lean protein, vegetables that are low starch, a healthy type fat and if you choose to, but it is not necessary, a starch such as a starchy vegetable or whole grain products.

You can mix and match to combine those elements into a great dinner, add a little bit of low fat sauce or some seasoning to your protein and you have a meal.

Lean proteins are the proteins that you need to eat, not fat heavy foods. If you are eating chicken, make sure that it is skinless.

Skinless chicken and turkey breast are versatile to cook with and you can cook some ahead so you always have some on hand that just needs warmed up for lunches and dinners both, a great way to save time on cooking.

You can substitute ground turkey for ground hamburger in any recipe to make your meal lower fat and lower calorie.

Turkey burgers and veggie patty burgers are great replacements for ground beef patties. For convenience, canned light tuna and canned salmon are great for lunches.

For dinners, you should eat halibut, cod, tilapia, and flounder as your fish choices. Shellfish that are good dinner choices are shrimp, scallops, crab-not imitation crab-oysters, and lobster; just go easy on the butter if you are dipping it in clarified butter.

Eggs or egg whites are great proteins that are lean. Tofu is a vegetarian option for protein and is versatile to cook with, especially in a stir-fry.

For red meat, your best choices are to eat pork, veal chops, Canadian bacon, lean ground beef, round roast, sirloin, tenderloin and rump roast cuts and lean ham.

Low starch vegetables are green beans, zucchini, summer squash, spinach, peppers, onions, mushrooms, eggplant, cucumber, celery, cauliflower, artichokes, broccoli, cabbage, collard greens, cauliflower, brussel sprouts, and asparagus.

You will find healthy fats in avocados-try some sliced on top of your salad-, canola oil, flaxseed oil, extra virgin olive oil, sesame oil, pumpkin seed oil, coconut oil, peanut oil, nuts, nut butters, and seeds. Use these healthier cooking oils for your cooking and add some seeds or nuts to your salad for some extra crunch or even as a coating for baking fish or chicken.

You can get your starch by eating products that are made with whole grains such as whole grain breads, whole grain pita bread, whole-wheat tortillas and wraps, whole-wheat pasta, barley, brown rice, oats, quinoa, and whole-wheat couscous.

Several vegetables are starchy and they belong in this category as well. Starchy vegetables include yams and sweet potatoes, winter squash, white potatoes, pumpkin, plantains, parsnips, green peas, corn, carrots, beets, and beans.

For your sauces and seasonings you can use the following, but use sparingly, BBQ sauces, mustard and stone ground mustard, fat-free salad dressing, horseradish, fresh salsa or pico de gallo, balsamic vinegar, red wine vinegar, marinara sauce, low sodium teriyaki, low sodium soy, fruit preserves-use only 100% fruit preserves, and fruit chutneys.

With those choices, you can assemble a variety of tasty and filling meals. If time is against you, buy a whole roasted chicken at the market, or pop a whole chicken in your crockpot along with some sliced potatoes and veggies, when you get home you will

have a great dinner. Same with the lean cuts of
meat, it all goes nicely with the crockpot and will fit
into your busy schedule.

Conclusion

When your days are full, finding time to get fit and to eat right is very hard; it does not matter if you are in the office all day, or a stay at home parent.

Losing weight just seems like something that is not in the cards because you simply have no time; however, you do have time, you just never realized how easy it was to make the changes that you need to make to lose weight and get more active.

It is possible. Dieting is not about what you do not eat, it is more about what you add to your diet, so that you are eating the right things and not the wrong ones.

Yes, you will need to cut out or limit several things, but if you are serious about losing weight and getting healthy, it is worth it.

Just by buying this book, you know that you are ready to commit and now that you know that you will be able to work around your schedule with ease, we hope you are excited about embarking upon this new path, the path to being healthy.

Exercise and diet combined is the best way to lose weight and you can achieve your exercise needs in just ten minutes a day six days a week, or thirty minutes a day three days a week at a minimum to boost your weight loss factor.

Now that you see how easy it is to work activities that get you fit into your day, you can even increase that amount to get faster results, it is your schedule, and now that you know the tools, you can apply them as you see fit.